DISCOVER THE
FOUNTAIN OF YOUTH

DISCOVER THE FOUNTAIN OF YOUTH

Velvet Fitzsimmons

To order additional copies of this book, contact:
Xlibris Corporation
1-888-795-4274
www.Xlibris.com
Orders@Xlibris.com
124131

Contents

Yes, you also can discover the fountain of youth.

This teaching manual will teach you how to become healthy as well as how to reverse the aging process.

You will also learn how to kill off cancer by simply drinking alkaline water as well as how to kill off the fungus in your body that may be making you sick.

Also lose weight simply by drinking alkaline water.

THE HUMAN BODY IS A VERY COMPLEX MACHINE.

THE HUMAN BRAIN COMPUTATES 100,000 AUDITORY AND 2,000,000 VISUAL INPUTS PER SECOND.

THUS, MAKING IT THE MOST REMARKABLE INSTRUMENT IN THE UNIVERSE!

THOUGH NO ONE CAN GO BACK
AND MAKE A BRAND NEW START,

ANYONE CAN START FROM NOW
AND MAKE A BRAND NEW END!

I am 46 years old.

In this booklet I will show you my secrets for looking and staying young. With the use of alkaline water, vitamin & mineral supplementation, and candida yeast therapy supplements, you too can become young and healthy again.

Step 1: I will discuss Alkaline water.

Alkaline water may also detoxify the body, and the anti-oxidant properties in it, can help to reverse the aging process.

Imagine growning healthier and younger with just a matter of changing the water that you drink!

Also, by drinking alkaline water, the candida yeast fungus that lives in our body may die off, thus promoting weight loss. Most people do not realize that weight gain may be pounds of fungus and not fat cells. This is one reason that people diet and don't lose weight, because fungus has to be killed off, and the only way to do this is with candida yeast fungus therapy.

When we are born our bodies are in an alkaline ph state. This means that our ph level is in balance. As we grow and our food and fluid intake changes, we often consume acidic foods and fluids that put our bodies in an acidic ph state. In an alkaline state diseases and illnesses do not thrive, and we stay healthy. In an acidic state, illnesses such as cancer, and other diseases thrive. So, if we put our bodies back into an alkaline ph state cancer cannot survive and it dies off. Imagine wiping out cancer just by changing the water that we drink!

The bottled water that we buy is all acidic. To test this on your own, go to a pool store and purchase a pool ph kit. Test the water for yourself. You will see that the botled water that you purchase is not healthy. In fact, it puts your body in an acidic state. Tap water is neutral ph. You would be better off to buy a water filter pitcher and purify your water this way than to buy bottled water. Also, when it comes to sodas, they are extremely acidic.

You would have to drink one and a half quarts of water to bring your ph balance back to neutral after drinking only one can soda.

It is now possible to purchase a home water machine that turns your water into alkaline water. Imagine never buying bottled water again. How great this would be for the environment without all those bottles in our landfills. GO GREEN!

To find out more about purchasing a home water machine for yourself, please call Velvet at: 478-396-7459. Alkaline water is also extremely healthy for your pets. Give them the gift of health as well as yourself.

Water truly is the fountain of youth, but you must drink the right kind. Start drinking alkaline water today and start your body on the road to better health. Alkaline water also reduces the pain and inflammation of diseases such as arthritis and fibromyalgia.

<u>Water is the major factor in these bodily functions:</u>

circulation
assimilation
digestion
elimination
temperature control

To ensure good health, dietary guidelines recommend that we drink eight glasses of water per day. Most of us don't, primarily because we don't like the taste of our tap water. Consider the importance of water to your well-being. Without water, our bodies simply cannot function, and it's no wonder. Our bodies are made up of about 70% water.

Do not take medications or vitamins with alkaline water. Use regular water or juice to take meds and vitamins with.

Step 2: I will discuss vitamin & mineral supplementation

Nutritional supplements

Vitamins influence the health and vibrancy of nearly every organ in the body! Vitamins may help forestall or even reverse many diseases including cancer, heart disease, osteoporosis, a weakening of the immune system, nerve degeneration, and other chronic disorders!

Articles documenting the importance of vitamins, minerals, and other supplements have been published in major medical and lay publications. Such supplements are especially appropriate for people with yeast-related health problems. You should only purchase yeast-free, sugar-free, color-free multivitamin, mineral, and antioxidant preparations.

You may have to rebuild your body from many years of nutritional deficiencies. I take a multivitamin every day. I also take a vitamin C and a vitamin E together every day. Vitamin C and vitamin E work synergistically. This means that they work better when taken together. This regimen tremendously affects the aging process. It slows it down and even reverses it. I also take a vitamin B supplement for my brain and central nervous system.

You should consult with your medical doctor before taking any vitamin supplements. Some vitamins and minerals may interfere with medications. Use caution, always ask your doctor for his or her advice.

Step 3: The Candida Yeast Syndrome and how to treat it.

Candida Albicans

Candida Albicans is a type of parasitic yeastlike fungus that inhabits the intestines, genital tract, mouth, esophagus, and throat. Normally this fungus lives in healthy balance with the other bacteria and yeasts in the body; however certain conditions can cause it to multiply, weakening the immune system and causing an infection known as candidiasis. The fungus can travel through the bloodstream to many parts of the body.

Because candidiasis can affect various parts of the body-the most common being the mouth, ears, nose, gastrointestinal tract, and vagina-it can be characterized by many symptoms. Symptoms often worsen in damp and/ or moldy places, and after the consumption of foods containing sugar and/ or yeast. Because of its many and varied symptoms, this disorder is often misdiagnosed.

When candida infects the vagina, it results in vaginitis characterized by a large amount of white, cheesy discharge and intense itching and burning, When the candida fungus infects the oral cavity, it is called thrush. White sores may form on the tongue, gums, and inside the cheeks. In a baby, the white spots of oral thrush may resemble milk spots. Oral thrush in an infant can spread to the mother's nipples and can lead to a situation in which mother and baby continually reinfect each other. Thrush may also infect a baby's buttocks, appearing as a diaper rash. Candida infection may also take the form of Athlete's foot or jock itch.

Systemic candidiasis is an overgrowth of candida everywhere, throughout the body. In the most severe cases, candida can travel through the bloodstream to invade every organ system in the body, causing a type of blood poisoning called candida septicemia. This condition almost always occurs in persons with serious underlying illnesses, such as advanced cancer or AIDS, and in persons with compromised immune systems. Anyone who has been on long-term antibiotic therapy, or has taken antibiotics often, probqably has an overgrowth of candida somewhere in his or her body. Antibiotics weaken the immune system and also destroy the "friendly bacteria" that normally keep candida yeasts under control. As it proliferates, the fungus releases toxins that weaken the immune system further.

Do you have any of these symptoms?

POSSIBLE YEAST-RELATED DISORDERS

constipation
autism
diarrhea
colitis
canker sores
abdominal pain
knotted muscles
bad breath
persistent heartburn
memory loss
mood swings
rectal itching
joint pain
acne
prostatitis
impotence
night sweats
clogged sinuses
pms
congestion
burning tongue
sneezing
post nasal drip
white spots on the tongue and in the mouth
chronic fatigue syndrome

nagging cough
shortness of breath
vaginitis
endometriosis
arthritis
pain down the back
hyperactivity
hormone imbalances
numbness in the face or extremities
kidney and bladder infections
a headache that never goes away
crave sugar
interstitial cystitis
irrational irritability
sleep disturbances
diabetes
hypoglycemia
irritability
adrenal problems
diarrhea
joint pain
psoriasis
chronic hives
eczema
anxiety
schizophrenia
brain disturbances
hearing loss
dizziness
digestive problems
bloating and/or gas
are bothered by food sensitivities
edema scleroderma
recurrent urinary tract infections
lupus
endocrine system disturbances
asthma
tightness in the chest
memory loss

feel "sick all over" or "feel poisoned"
rheumatoid arthritis
have sought help from many different specialists
mood swings
sensitivity to tobacco smoke, perfumes, and other chemicals
multiple chemical sensitivity syndrome
sexual dysfunction and/or infertility
have taken a lot of antibiotic drugs
multiple sclerosis
have taken birth control pills and/or steroids
sometimes feel spaced out
central nervous system disturbances
headaches and/or migraines
muscle aches and/or muscle pain
sore throat
hormone imbalances
myasthenia gravis
chrohn's disease
stiffness in the neck and/or shoulder area
hypothyroidism
tingling sensations
inability to cope
inability to function in the home or workplace
pain or pressure in the jaw

Yeast-What they are and how they make you sick.

Yeasts are single cell living organisms, which are neither animal nor vegetable. They live on the surfaces of all living things, including fruits, vegetables, grains, and your skin. They are a part of the "microflora" which contribute in various ways to the health of its host. Yeast is a kind of fungus. Mildew, mold, mushrooms, monilla, and candida are all names that are used to describe different types of yeast. And one family of yeasts, candida albicans, normally lives on the inner warm creases of the digestive tract and vagina. Yeasts have some very animal-like behavior and they must consume other substances such as sugar and fats in order to survive. In addition, candida albicans has been referred to as a "Dr. Jekyll and Mr. Hyde" sort of critter. Here's why: it can branch from a single cell yeast form into a branching fungal form. And these branches can burrow beneath the surfaces of your mucous membranes. This branching fungal form. This branching fungal form may then spread out like a spiderweb to engulf the entire body. This is especially noticeable around the ocular eye orbit where the skin is thin. Darkened circles under the eyes and many times the entire area around the eye may appear darkened and even black.

Why you may develop yeast-related health problems.

The common yeast, candida albicans, normally lives in your body, especially in the vagina and intestines. When your immune system is strong candida yeasts cause no problems. But when you take broad-spectrum antibiotics for an infection, these drugs kill our friendly germs while they're killing the enemies. These antibiotics do not affect candida yeasts. And since there is no friendly bacteria in the intestines, the bad bacteria, the candida yeasts get all the food and nutrition that you take in. So they multiply and raise large families of yeasts. These candida yeasts put out toxins that weaken your immune system. So you may experience repeated infections. Each infection is treated with antibiotics. So a vicious cycle develops. Once these friendly bateria have been knocked out even once with the use of antibiotics it is possible that you may have a yeast overgrowth in your body.

Other causes of yeast overgrowth include:

Hormonal changes associated with the normal menstrual cycle, birth control pills, pregnancy, steroids by pill, injection, or inhalation, genital irritations and abrasions, re-infection from your sexual partner, diabetes, and sugar rich diets.

How yeast affects the body.

Remember that yeast have some animal like behavior characteristics. This means that it must eat in order to live and continue surviving in the body. Like an animal, without a food source, it dies. When you eat and drink, what you take in goes to the stomach where it is broken down into simple substances that the body can absorb. It then moves on into the intestines. The majority of food would naturally be absorbed straight into the intestinal wall and then be distributed throughout the body via the bloodstream. This is how the cells get the needed energy to run and maintain the body and to sustain life.

However, remember that candida yeast has some animal like behavior characteristics. How does a hungry animal eat? Ravenously! The yeast reaches out and engulfs the food before your body has a chance to engulf it. Your body cells are then left without the proper nutrition needed to function and perform properly. This sets off system disturbances that cause symptoms to appear in all sorts of varied places throughout the body. Also, as the yeast eat, they produce waste that contain powerful toxins and poisons.

Candida overgrowth in the intestinal tract may create what has been called a "leaky gut". As a result, food antigens and toxins may pass through this membrane and be distributed throughout the body via the bloodstream. This can give you a feeling of being "sick all over". Any one of these poisons can damamge a cell and cause it to reproduce out of control. Physicians's diagnose a cell reproducing out of control as "cancer". These poisons and toxins also weaken the immune system. In fact, research has reported that the candida yeast causes a reduction in the body's T4 cell. This cell is the main diagnosing factor in the AIDS virus.

As the yeast grows not only do all of the cells of the body become malnourished from a lack of nutrition and oxygen, your cells start getting squashed from the pressure of the yeast pressing down upon your cells. This inflicts severe disturbances in the nervous system, which controls all of our nerve impulses and transmissions. This yeast may even produce symptoms that mimic multiple sclerosis and manic depression.

Many of the yeast-related symptoms especially headache, depression, and mood swings, develop because the immune system, the endocrine system, and the brain are intimately related. And although we sometimes forget, every part of the body is connected to every other part!

Steps to regain your health!

If your health problems are yeast connected, a special diet and antifungal medication will start you on the road to recovery. Candida-related illness is never an illness unto itself. Persons who suffer from almost any dysfunction related to candida always have food intolerances and these may be severe. Generally sugar in any form is the most consequential offender. Candida-related illness must always be treated, at least initially with stringent dietary control in antifungal therapy. There is practically no hope of succssful treatment of this problem without dietary restriction.

Clean up your diet!

If you want to overcome your yeast-related health problems, you must change your diet! As a first step-go to your kitchen and get rid of the sugar, corn syrup, white bread, and other white flour products, soft drinks, and most ready-to-eat cereals. Foods and beverages containing these nutritionally deficient simple carbohydrates promote poor health. To overcome a candida-related health problem, you'll need to avoid them.

To replace sugar you can use liquid saccharin (sweeta or fasweet) or fructooligosaccharides (FOS), which you can find at some pharmacies and health food stores. Replace them with more vegetables, including some you don't usually eat. Also, go to your health food store and buy some of the "grain alternatives"-Amaranth, quinoa, and buckwheat. These nutritious foods are rich in carbohydrates and help fill you up. They are also useful for people who are sensitive to wheat and corn.

You will also need to get rid of foods containing hydrogenated oils (especially coconut and other tropical oils) and replace them with modest amounts of unrefined oils, including flaxseed, canola, and olive.

Avoid yeasty foods and beverages, especially dried fruits, mushrooms, condiments, alcohol, juices (except for freshly squeezed juices), leavened breads, bagels, pastries, pizza, and rolls. In two or three weeks after you improve, you can try a yeasty food and see if it bothers you.

Diets aren't forever and after a few weeks, or months, you may be able to relax a bit. Yet, until you show significant improvement, stick to your diet.

The best diet to begin with.

Low-sugar, low-yeast-, dairy-free.

Food sensitivities are present in almost every person with candida-related health problems. They play a major role in causing symptoms, so they must be identified and properly managed. Any food may cause an adverse reaction!

FATS

Fats are an important constituent of foods and are found in almost every part of your body. Like carbohydrates, they are sources of metabolic energy. They help move the fat-soluble vitamins across the walls of your intestines and into your bloodstream.

Although fats are present in foods of all kinds, they're found especially in animal products, including meat, dairy products and eggs. Most fats contain relatively few vitamins, minerals, or fiber. So the calories in these foods are often labeled "empty calories". Also, many animals are given antibiotics. When you consume these antibiotic-laden foods, they may cause alterations in the balance in the normal bacteria in your intestinal tract. Along with these alterations, candida albicans may proliferate (multiply).

Farm animals are often injected with hormones. When their flesh or milk is consumed, these hormones enter our body. Finally, animals consume insecticides and other toxic chemicals and concentrate (store) them in their fat tissues. So when we eat animal products, we take on poisonous toxin and chemical substances called "xenobiotics". Even lean meat, chicken, and fish contain high concentrations of these xenobiotic chemicals.

Some physicians feel that these chemicals have been responsible for the appearnance of new man-made diseases.

So to reduce your fat intake, sharply limit or avoid these foods. Also, dairy products create mucous in the body. Remember that yeasts live in the underlying burrows of mucous membranes. <u>Avoid the dairy!</u>

You should not avoid all fats because there are good ones as well as bad ones. The good ones are called essential fatty acids (EFA's). You need them to enjor good health.

Essential Fatty Acids (EFA's)

Essential Fatty Acids (EFA's), including flaxseed oil. Flax is one of the world's oldest known cultivated plants and is beneficial in the treatment of PMS and all major degenerative disease. These include MS, cancer, heart disease, and arthritis. <u>Flaxseed oil</u> is the richest source of the polyunsaturated essential fatty acid, linolenic acid. It is richest known source of omega 3 fatty acids for vegetarians.

Flaxseeds are the major source of <u>omega 3 fatty acids</u>. They also contain other oils, including <u>omega 6 essentail fatty acids</u>. You can mix it with lemon juice and use it for salad dressing, or take it "straight". The usual dose is one to two tablespoons per day. You can also buy flaxseeds and grind them to a powder. Because flax oil can become rancid, it should be dispensed in dark glass bottles and kept refrogerated. The bottles should be dated as well, as it has a short shelf life of only three to four months at most. Omega 3 oils may also be purchased in capsules. They too, can become rancid after a time, so be sure to monitor the date on your supply.

Along with the flax oil supplement you should eat more vegetables and avoid sugar, alcohol, and the bad fats (hydrogenated vegetable oils and saturated fats). Vitamin C, B3, B6, zinc, and magnesium are required if a person is to fully utilize and enjoy the benefits of flaxseed oil.

Oils which are especially rich in omega 6 EFA's include evening primrose oil (Efamol), Borage, and Black Currant seed oils. These oils are especially recommended for women with PMS and certain types of eczema.

Oil of Evening Primrose is a rich source of a particular omega 6 fatty acid. Benefits of supplementation with this oil include: relieving premenstrual breast pain and other symtpms of PMS; preventing atrophy of the lacrimal (tear producing) glands, stopping nerve deterioration in MS; and improving certain kinds of eczema. Symptoms that showed improvement included dizziness, vertigo, depression, memory loss, exhaustion, muscle weakness, aches, pain, and loss of concentration.

EFA's are found in plants and their seeds, including flax, walnut, sunflower, safflower, corn, canola, and evening primrose. They are also found in the fat of cold water fish, including salmon, mackerel, sardines, tuna, and herring. Like vitamins, EFA's cannot be manufactured in the body and so must be supplied in the diet. EFA's perform many vital functions within the body.

They furnish raw materials for making hormones, including the prostaglandins, the short-distance message carriers that are made by all the cells of the body. They form the structural wall of each of the body's cells. The body has billions of cells of various sizes, shapes, and functions. Each cell has around it a waterproof boundary that is made of oils. Numerous membranes inside the cell where the cell's "business" takes place are also made of oils. It is estimated that if you took all of the cells of the human body and laid them out on a flat surface, it would cover about ten football fields. Flexibility of these membranes, which is critical to their proper functioning, is imparted by the benefit of the EFAs. Essential fatty acids come directly and only from the food we eat. In no other way is the expression "You are what you eat" more accurate.

Candida yeast can cause metabolic disturbances including a disturbance in proteins, carbohydrates, and essential fatty acids (omega 3 and omega 6).

Benefits of EFAs

EFAs are good for you. They help to prevent and treat high cholesterol, high blood pressure, and cardiovascular disease.
Balance is the key to healthy nutrition. Omega 3 and Omega 6 are essential fatty acids. A balance of oils and foods rich in these EFAs help prevent and treat disease. Very low-fat diets can be harmful and should not be used by people trying to lose weight. The cholesterol content of food has

relatively little impact on cholesterol levels. Rather, it is excess saturated fat and calories which cause your body to make more cholesterol.

It is best not to use either butter or margarine. If you need to put some fat on your bread or vegetables, try a little oil like the Italians and Greeks, who have the lowest coronary heart disease risk.

Simple Carbohydrates

(sugar)

Yeasts thrive on simple carbohydrates. These include cane sugar, beet sugar, honey, corn syrup, maple syrup, and molasses. Research has shown that this form of sugar can enable the candida yeast to multiply as much as 200 times.

Aviod this form of sugar! This is a vicious cycle that occurs every time you eat this sugar. Eat this sugar, yeast grows! This sugar is the main form of food for the candida yeast. Every time you satisfy a sugar craving you are feeding this yeast! Don't do it! Your very health may depend upon it!

In addition, eating fruits promotes yeast growth. Here's why. Fruits are loaded with fructose. In spite of their fiber content, fruits are readily converted to fructose and other simple sugars in the intestinal tract, thereby encouraging the growth of candida albicans. Fruits are usually eliminated from the diet for the first 3 weeks.

Limiting the intake of sweets and starches deprives candia yeast of the nutrient that allows its maximun multiplication.

Fructooligosaccharides (FOS)

"FOS" are sucrose molecules to which 1, 2, or 3 additional fructose molecules have been linked in sequence. FOS are widely distributed in a variety of edible plants such as vegetables and grains and some fruits. They are not absorbed by human digestive enzymes in the gastrointestinal tract, but are utilized by your friendly intestinal bacteria.

"FOS" promotes the growth of beneficial bacteria including Lactobacilli and Bifidus. And in doing so they interfere with the growth of disease-causing organisms.

"FOS" occur in small amounts in nature. In onion, garlic, burdock, bananas, wheat, rye, barley, oats, and a few other vegetables and fruits. Commercially produced FOS appears to be identical to those from natural sources.

"FOS" is a polysaccharide-very sweet. It is so complex that yeast cannot utilize it all, yet other bacteria can. If you ingest it into the digestive tract, it makes the friendly bacteria grow like crazy! This makes good sense because what you are really trying to do is repopulate your colon with good bacteria.

Benefits of "FOS"

Proliferation of good bacteria producing a reduction of detrimental bacteria
Reduction of toxic metabolites and detrimental enzymes
Prevention of pathogenic and autogenic diarrhea
Prevention of constipation
Protection of liver function
Reduction of serum cholesterol
Anticancer effect
Production of nutrients

How does "FOS" compare to sugar?

It is perhaps half as sweet.

Aspartame

Aspartame is responsible for many distressing medical problems, ranging from headaches and memory loss to hyperactivity in children and seizure disorders.

Aspartame is now consumed by more than 100 million persons in the United States. The consumption of aspartame has increased at an astonishing rate since 1981, when this man-made sweetener was first introduced. By 1985, 800 million pounds of aspartame was used per year in the United States.

Equally important, the public, increasingly concerned in recent years about all food additives, has been reassured that aspartame is entirely safe and can be used without worry.

MIT lab tests showing that aspartame, the principle ingredient in nutrasweet, destroys neurotransmitters, the chemicals that convey messages between neurons within the brain.

Research has shown that artificial sweeteners may interfere with obtaining adequate nutrients essential for good health. And, rather than helping people lose weight, they may actually promote weight gain!

Complex Carbohydrates

(Plant Foods)

Complex carbohydrates, especially vegetables, play a critically important role in enabling you to enjoy good health. Plant foods contain enough calories to meet the energy requirements of the active person. They contain plenty of protein (including all the essential amino acids), essential fats, fibers, and minerals required to meet people's daily dietary needs.

Vegetarian foods in their natural form are primarily complex carbohydrates. For example, grains, beans, vegetables, fruits, and so on. Complex carbohydrates are very filling. In contrast, simple carbohydrates are "empty calories". That is, calories without any nutritional value. So it's easy to eat a lot of calories without being aware of it. Besides being more filling than simple sugars, complex carbohydrates are hard for your body to convert into fat.

Increase the amount of carbohydrates consumed to where you've doubled the amount of calories you get from carbohydrate foods, especially those rich in fiber and low in refined sugar. To do this, eat more fruits, vegetables, legumes, and whole grains.

A high-complex diet will not only help you feel better and improve your present health, it will also lessen your chances of developing heart disease as you grow older.

<u>Health benefits of complex carbohydrates</u>

They promote friendly intestinal bacteria that may counteract candida
    overgrowth.
They provide vitamins, minerals, and antioxidants.
They provide fiber, promoting normal elimination, lessening your chances
    of absorbing food allergens and other toxins.
They promote the absorption and retention of calcium, lessening your
    chances of developing osteoporosis.
They promote the release of glucose to meet your energy needs.

Plants contain phytochemicals (these are the substances that give fruit, vegetables, and plants, their color and flavor characteristics). These phytochemicals seem to be able to throw a biological wrench into one or more of the mechanisms leading to a tumor. At almost every one of the steps along the pathway leading to cancer, there are one or more compounds in fruits or vegetables that will slow up or reverse the process! Plant foods also contain lots of antioxidant nutrients which protect people against free radical buildup.

If you want to be healthy, you should consume a lot more fiber. It promotes a "rapid transit time" through the intestinal tract. As a result, the healthy person will pass two to three loose bowel movements per day. If you want to remain healthy, let the waste pass through you promptly.

Proteins

Our immune defense system requires protein, especially for the formation of antibodies that help fight infections. Hemoglobin, our oxygen-carrying, red-blood-cell molecule is a protein, as are many hormones that regulate our metabolism, such as thyroid and insulin. Protein is needed for the growth of body tissues; it is vitally important during childhood, pregnancy, and lactation.

Amino acids are the building blocks of protein. We must obtain these from food, but not necessarily from meat. In fact, we're able to use the amino acids obtained from vegetable sources very efficiently. It is virtually impossible to develop a protein deficiency on a vegetarian diet.

The average American gets 2/3 of his or her protein from meat, fish, dairy, poultry, and eggs. Only 1/3 comes from plants (beans, legumes, and grains mostly). Unfortunately, most animal protein carries a hefty price tag, artery-clogging, saturated fat and cholesterol. You don't need any animal protein to be healthy!

You can eliminate milk, eggs, and all animal protein from your diet and still be healthy in your adult years. Complete vegetarians, get their calcium from broccoli, kale, collards, and other plant foods, (and all the protein they need in beans and whole grains).

A high-protein diet can be harmful to persons suffering from kidney disease.

Foods we should eat every day.

8 or more servings of whole grains, including whole wheat bread, pasta, cereals, and brown rice.

6 or more servings of vegetables, including dark green and leafy vegetables, sweet potatoes, squash, cabbage, and brussel sprouts.

4 or more servings of fruits, including citrus fruits, papaya, strawberries, mango, apricot, and cantaloupe.

2 or 3 servings of dried beans and tofu.

2 or 3 servings of calcium-rich foods such as collard greens, kale, seaweed, and non-fat milk or yogurt.

Up to 4 tablespoons of monosaturated oils, such as canola and olive oil.

Truly yeast-free diets are impossible to come by. Yeast and other molds are ubiquitous on the surfaces of fruits, vegetables, and grains. They can only be avoided completely by eating only fresh dairy, meat, fish, and peeled fruits and vegetables. So, from a practical standpoint, the complete avoidance of yeasts and molds in ones diet is really not feasible.

Foods to avoid

Leavened foods (breads, bagels, pastries, pretzels, crackers, pizza dough, and rolls), fermented and aged products, including alcohol, cheeses, commercially prepared juices, dried fruits, condiments, sauces and mushrooms, milk, yeast, chocolate, soft drinks, sugar, punches, citrus, wheat, corn, processed and packaged foods, and food coloring and additives.

Avoid Alcohol!! All alcoholic beverages are loaded with yeast. Alcohol contains large amounts of quick acting carbohydrates which make yeast multiply like crazy!!

Non-prescription anti-yeast agents

Probiotics-Probiotics are a group of friendly bacteria that help us stay well. They include lactobacillus acidophilus and bifidobacteria. These bacteria have been used by physicians and non-physicians to treat complaints ranging from constipation and diarrhea to skin problems. Preparations of live lactobacilli may be especially helpful if taken every day.

Inside each of us live vast numbers of bacteria without which we could not remain in good health. There ae several thousand billion in each person. Most of them living in the digestive tract. If they were all placed together the total weight of these "friendly" bacteria would come to nearly four pounds. These bacteria perform many important functions in the body. However, not all of the friendly bacteria perform the same functions, some being far more useful and plentiful than others. Certain bacteria help to maintain good health, while others have a definite value in helping us to regain health once it haas been upset.

These dual protective and therapeutic roles help explain why the word "probiotics" was coined, since it means "for life". The most important criteria for activity of probiotic substances is that there must be an adequate number of live organisms. You may find probiotic products in a health food store. Lactobacillus acidophilus is an excellent source of live lactobacilli bacteria.

<u>Citrus seed extracts</u>-These extracts are as effective as nystatin and caprylic acid in treating persons with yeast overgrowth in the intestinal tract. They are also useful in treating persons with Giardiasis and other intestinal parasites.

<u>Caprylic acid</u> is an excellent candida yeast fungus killer and is available at health food stores.

The liquid preparations must be diluted and stirred well in at least 4 ounces of water. If taken undiluted, this product will irritate your mucous membranes.

A qualified physician should check anyone who has a candida yeast-related health problem for intestinal parasites.

<u>Garlic cloves or kyolic</u>-kyolic is aged garlic, and has been proven to be very effective in the treatment of candida. Garlic is also a blood thinner and has been proven useful in the treatment of lowering high blood pressure. Please <u>consult your physician </u>before taking this natural herb.

Your physician may prescribe prescription yeast medications. They include Nystatin, Nizoral, Diflucan, Sporanox, Lamisil, and Amphotericin B.

Lifestyle changes

You'll need fresh air, sunlight (or skylight), exercise and a proper amount of sleep. Don't be a "couch potato" who spends hours looking at the television. Take a walk, do calisthenics and play outdoor games. Get plenty of exercise!

Psychological support

You'll need emotional and psychological nutrients, whether you are sick or well. Here are a few of them: encouragement, love, praise, touch, hugs, and laughter. They will strengthen your immune system and play an important role in helping you to overcome your health problems. Of course, prayer and faith provide the best means of emotional and strengthening support.

Control chemical exposures

Almost without exception, people with yeast-related health problems are sensitive to chemicals they come in contact with during everyday life. These include tobacco smoke, colognes, glues, carpet odors, paints, formaldehyde, insecticides, diesel fumes, and other traffic odors.

The yeast are microscopic bacteria, they feed off odors in the air. The nausea feeling that people sometimes get when they come in contact with odors is actually the candida yeast multiplying in the intestinal tract. Although you cannot avoid all these things, you can "clean up your home". By getting rid of odorous bathroom and kitchen chemicals, insecticides and other volatile inhalants your symptoms should start improving very quickly. Also, do what you can to clean up your workplace.

You may also react to chemicals in and on your food, even fresh foods, as well as those found in cans, plastic wrappings and other food containers. So where possible, purchase and eat organic foods and choose prepared foods in glass containers.

Chemical exposures adversely affect many parts of your immune system. Chemicals you're exposed to resemble pipes draining into a rain barrel. The barrel represents a resistance. If you continue to be exposed to chemicals, the barrel overflows and you develop symptoms.

Infections of various types, including viral and yeast infections, may also precipitate a "leak" in your barrel, even when the barrel isn't full. In time, our fat stores can become saturated with the smorgasbord of chemicals that we eat, drink, or absorb through our skin. Some chemicals cannot be completely broken down and removed by means of our expired air, perspiration, saliva, urine, and bowel movements.

Once these chemicals enter the body, they pass easily into the brain, which is the most lipid organ of the body. The most common brain symptoms include depression, inability to think straight, exhaustion, dizziness, and headache.

We must wonder how long our bodies, as well as those of our children, can handle our progressively increasing chemical overload.

We are the first generation in the history of the world that has been exposed over a lifetime to synthetic and toxic chemicals in our food, air, water, and products we use. Before 1940 everyone lived on organic foods; pesticides weren't invented yet.

There were no toxic waste dumps, preservatives in food, antibiotics, malathion spray, chlorinated water, tight buildings, aerosol sprays, synthetic carpeting, formaldehyde products, or major cosmetics and perfume industries.

The AIDS epidemic, sexual permissiveness, the birth control pill, widespread legal and illegal drug use, sedentary living, and convenience foods have changed the way we live. We are a more vulnerable population, not as biologically strong!

Since 1950 we've seen the development and overuse of antibiotics; the use of hormones and birth control pills; the development of immunosuppressive drugs; the introduction of various chemical and toxins into our environment; and significant changes which have occurred within our diets, leaving us foods tainted with pesticides, depleted in nutritional value, and loaded with sugars and dyes.

All these things have interfered with our body's life chemistry, our "biochemistry". Cells then degerate, and these degenerative processes manifest as degenerative diseases.

Can we really believe that these changes have not affected the well-being of some, and eventually, perhaps all of us?

WITH PERMISSION: RESEARCHED AND COMPILED FROM THE BOOK "THE YEAST CONNECTION" BY WILLIAM G. CROOK M.D. FOUNDER OF THE INTERNATIONAL WORLD HEALTH ORGANIZATION LOCATED IN JACKSON, TN.

Nutrients Defined

REFERENCES:

"PRESCRIPTION FOR NUTRITIONAL HEALING" BY
JAMES F. BALCH MD. & PHYLLIS A. BALCH C.N.C.

ANTIOXIDANTS-There is a group of vitamins, minerals, and enzymes called antioxidants that help protect the body from the formation of free radicals. Free radicals are atoms or groups of atoms that can cause damage to cells, impairing the immune system and leading to infections and various degenerative disorders such as head and brain diseases and cancer. Free radical damage is thought by scientists to be the basis for the aging process as well. There are a number of known free radicals that occur in the body. They may be formed by exposure to radiation and toxic chemicals, such as those found in cigarette smoke, overexposure to the sun's rays, or various metabolic processes, such as the process of breaking down stored fat molecules for use as an energy source. Free radicals are normally kept in check by the action of the radical scavengers that occur naturally in the body. These scavengers neutralize the free radicals. Certain enzymes serve this vital function. The body makes these, of course. There are also a number of nutrients that act as antioxidants, including vitamins A, C & E, beta-carotene, selenium, and the hormone melatonin which is a powerful free radical neutralizer. A high intake of antioxidant nutrients appears to be protective against cancer.

VITAMIN A/BETA-CAROTENE-Vitamin A is a retinol found in foods of animal origin. Beta-carotene-Provitamin A (provided by foods of both plant and animal origin. Found not to have the same toxicity level of Vitamin A (retinol). Vitamin A requires fats as well as minerals to be properly absorbed by your digestive tract. Vitamin A can be stored in the body and does not need replenishing every day. Slows the aging process. Counteracts night blindness. Promotes growth, strong bones,

31

healthy skin and hair. Aids in the proper functioning of the immune
system. Helps build resistance to respiratory infections. Deficiency
may cause night blindness, conjuctivitis, xerophthalmia, corneal
ulcers, infertility, birth defects, depressed immune system, bone
disease, poor growth in children, acne, dermatitis, hyperkeratosis
("goose flesh"), and an increased risk of cancer. Causes of depletion:
Contraceptives, cortisone, prednisone, alcohol, estrogen, mineral oil,
most drugs, coffee, air, pollutants, interior lighting.

VITAMIN B1 (thiamin)-Water soluble-excess is excreted and not stored
in the body. Must be replaced daily. Increases needed during illness,
surgery, and stress. Promotes growth. Improves your mental attitude.
Aids in digestion, especially of carbohydrates. Keeps the nervous
system, muscles, and heart functioning normally. Helps fight air or
seasickness. Relieves dental postoperative pain. Deficiency may cause
congestive heart failure, memory loss, anxiety, depression, lethargy,
muscle cramps, paralysis, emotional instability, loss of appetite, in
extreme cases beriberi (mostly in alcoholics). Causes of depletion:
Negative emotions, alcohol, cooking heat, caffeine, excess sugar,
tobacco, raw fish and shell fish, muscle relaxants, and sulfa drugs.

VITAMIN B2 (riboflavin)-Water soluble. Must be replaced daily. Is easily
absorbed, and is not destroyed by heat or oxidation. Helps eliminate
sore mouth, lips, and tongue. Benefits vision, alleviates eye fatigue.
Functions with other substances to metabolize carbohydrates, fats, and
proteins. Deficiency may cause cracks and sores around the mouth
and nose, problems with vision, and difficulty swallowing. Causes
of depletion: Alcohol, birth control pills, coffee, radiation, tobacco,
ultraviolet light, drugs, estrogen and sugar.

VITAMIN B3 (niacinamide, niacin)-Water-soluble. Body can manufacture
niacin from tryptophan, if it is not deficient in vitamins B1, B2, B6.
Essential for the synthesis of sex hormones (estrogen, progesterone,
testosterone) as well as cortisone, throxine, and insulin. Aids in
promoting a healthy digestive system. Increases energy through the
proper utilization of food. Can ease some attacks of diarrhea. Helps
prevent and ease the severity of migraine headaches. Increases
circulation and can reduce high blood pressure. Reduces cholesterol
and triglycerides. Necessary for a healthy nervous system and brain
functions. Deficiency may cause diarrhea, mouth sores, pellagra (a
skin disease). Niacin may cause flushing and niacinamide will not.

Causes of depletion: Caffeine, antibiotics, alcohol, sleeping pills, estrogen sugar, sulfa drugs.

VITAMIN B5 (pantothenic acid, panthenol)-Water-soluble. A member of the B-complex family. Essential for the conversion of fat and sugar to energy. Fight infection by building antibodies. Helps with treatment of postoperative shock. Vital for proper functioning of the adrenal glands. Can reduce adverse and toxic effects of many antibiotics. Deficiency may cause hypoglycemia, duodenal ulcers, blood and skin disorders. Causes of depletion: Insecticidal fumigants, alcohol, caffeine, cooking heat, sulfa drugs, estrogen and sleeping pills.

VITAMIN B6 (pyridoxine)-Water-soluble-excess is excreted and not stored in the body. Must be replaced daily. Helps to properly assimilate protein and fat. Aids in the conversion of tryptophan to niacin. Helps prevent various nervous and skin disorders. Promotes the proper synthesis of antiaging nucleic acids. Helps alleviate nausea. Reduces muscle and leg cramps, hand numbness and certain forms of neuritis in the extremities. Works as a natural diuretic. Deficiency may cause depression, mental confusion, inflammation of the mucous membranes of the mouth, patches of itchy, scaling skin, convulsions in infants, and anemia. Causes of depletion: Alcohol, oral contraceptives, estrogen, most drugs, and stress.

VITAMIN B12 (cyanocabalamin)-Water soluble. Must be replaced daily. Effective in very small doses. Not well assimilated through the stomach. Calcium helps to achieve proper benefits. Regenerates red blood cells, thereby preventing anemia. Promotes growth and increases appetite in children. Increases energy. Helps to maintain a healthy nervous system. Helps the body to properly utilize fats, carbohydrates and proteins. Helps relieve irritability. Improves concentration, memory and balance. Deficiency may cause pernicious anemia and neurological disorders. Causes of depletion: Laxatives, alcohol, antibiotics, aspirin, diuretics, antacids, tobacco, caffeine, estrogen, sleeping pills, contraceptives, intestinal parasites, cooking.

VITAMIN C-(ASCORBIC ACID)-Water-soluble. Has a primary role in the formation of collagen, which is important for the growth and repair of body tissue cells, gums, blood vessels, bones, and teeth. Heals wounds, burns, and bleeding gums. Can help accelerate healing after surgery. Aids in preventing many types of viral and bacterial infections and stimulates the immune system. Offers production against cancer-producing agents. Helps counteract the formation of nitrosamines (cancer-causing substances). Lowers the incidence of blood clots in veins. Aids in the treatment and prevention of the common cold. Prevents scurvy. Recommended as a preventive for SIDS (sudden infant death syndrome). Deficiency may cause bleeding gums, easy bruising, and slow healing. Causes of depletion: Alcohol, air pollution, cigarette smoking, birth control pills, antibiotics, stress, aspirin, pain killers, diuretics, cortisone. Because the body cannot manufacture vitamin C, it must be obtained in the diet or through the use of supplements. Unfortunately, most of the vitamin C consumed in the diet is lost in the urine.

VITAMIN D-(Calciferol)-Fat-soluble. Acquired through sunlight or diet. After suntan is established, vitamin D production through the skin stops. Essential for the health of the glandular and nervous system. It's main function is to regulate all mineral and vitamin metabolism especially calcium, phosphorous, and vitamin A. Taken with vitamins A and C can help prevent colds. Very important in childhood for healthy bone formation. Required for healthy nervous system maintenance. Good for skin, teeth, blood clotting, and a healthy thyroid gland. Deficiency may cause Rickets in children, bone softening in adults, insomnia, osteoporosis, tooth decay, muscle weakness, poor calcium absorption. Causes of depletion: Mineral oil, smog, barbiturates, Prednisone, Dilantin, sleeping pills, cortisone, anticonvulsant medications.

VITAMIN E (Tocopherol)-Fat-soluble and stored in organs and fatty tissues. 60 to 70 percent of daily doses are excreted in feces. Unlike other fat-soluble vitamins, vitamin E is stored in the body for a relatively short period of time. Slows aging, protects red blood cells. Prevents blood clots. Supplies oxygen to the body to give you more endurance. Aids in the prevention of miscarriages. Plays an essential role in cellular respiration of all muscles, especially cardiac and skeletal muscles. Maintains healthy muscles and nerves. Good for the hair and skin. Helps with burns and scars. Protects the lungs against air pollution by working with vitamin A. Caution: You should not take iron at the same time as vitamin E. Deficiency may cause the destruction of red blood cells, muscle degeneration, some anemia's and reproductive disorders, dry dull hair, sterility, miscarriages, heart disease, enlarged prostate. Causes of depletion: Estrogen, birth control pills, chlorine, mineral oil, heat, food processing, inorganic iron, rancid fat. Zinc is necessary to maintain proper levels of vitamin E in the blood.

VITAMIN K-Fat-soluble. Made by intestinal bacteria. Helps in preventing internal bleeding and hemorrhages. Promotes proper blood clotting. Aids in reducing excessive menstrual flow. May play a role in bone formation and help prevent osteoporosis. Necessary for normal liver functioning. Deficiency may cause a tendency to hemorrhage (bleed) resulting from prolonged blood clotting time, intestinal malabsorption, nose bleeding, miscarriage, diarrhea, cellular disease.

ALFALFA-Has been dubbed "the great healer" by European physicians. Excellent source of vitamins A, K, B6, E, D, & U. Contains eight essential enzymes and several minerals. Alkalizes and detoxifies the body. Promotes pituitary gland function. Balances hormones. Improves appetite. Reduces blood cholesterol levels and plaque deposits on artery walls. Good for colon disorders, ulcers, arthritis, hemorrhaging and bleeding-disorders, and diabetes. Contains an antifungus agent.

BEE PROPOLIS-Excellent aid against bacterial infections. Helps stimulate the immune system. May also help tonsillitis, ulcers, and halitosis. May reduce inflammation of the throat and mouth. Helps with dry cough and throat. May help with acne.

BIOFLAVONOIDS-(RUTIN, HESPERIDIN)-Water soluble, composed of citrin, rutin, hesperidin, as well as flavones and flavonals. Prevents vitamin C from being destroyed by oxidation. Strengthens the walls of capillaries, thereby preventing bruising. Helps build resistance to infection. Aids in preventing and healing bleeding gums. Anti-inflammatory and natural diuretic. Increases the effectiveness of vitamin C. Helps in the treatment of edema and dizziness due to disease of the inner ear. Deficiency may cause capillary fragility. Causes of depletion: Smoking, aspirin, alcohol, antibiotics, cortisone, pain killers.

BIOTIN-Water-soluble, sulfur containing, member of the B-complex family. Can be sensitized by intestinal bacteria. Essential for the normal metabolism of fat and protein. Essential for proper body chemistry. Aids in preventing graying hair. Helps in the prevention of baldness. Helps ease muscle pains. Alleviates eczema and dermatitis. Deficiency may cause eczema of the face and body, extreme exhaustion, impairment of fat metabolism, anorexia, alopecia, depression, insomnia.

BLUE COHOSH-Helps with menstrual disorders and cramps. Can help with anxiety and nervous disorders. Has anti-inflammatory properties so can help with arthritis. Has been found to have some antibiotic and immune-stimulating properties. Stimulates uterine contraction for childbirth and has been used to induce labor. May also help with coughs and asthma. Caution: People with high blood pressure, heart disease, glaucoma, or history of stroke should take caution when using this. PREGNANT WOMEN SHOULD NOT TAKE THIS!

BORON-Builds muscle tissue. Beneficial in the treatment of arthritis and post menopausal osteoporosis in women. Needed for calcium uptake and healthy bones. Maintains healthy cell membranes.

BURDOCK-Purifies the blood, restores liver and gallbladder function and stimulates the immune system. Some believe can help reduce cancer tumors. Can be used as a blood purifier, diuretic, and as a mild laxative. Can aid in treating skin disorders like acne, boils, carbuncles, and others. Can help with urinary tract infections, kidney problems, and painful urination. Caution: Pregnant women should not take this. It can be a uterine stimulant.

CALCIUM-Helps maintain strong bones and healthy teeth. Required for the maintenance of a regular heartbeat. Alleviates insomnia. Regulates the contraction and relaxation of muscles. Helps your body to metabolize iron. Aids the nervous system in the transmission of nerve impulses. Helps activate the enzymes that are needed to convert food into energy. May help prevent colon cancer. Essential in blood clotting. Deficiency may cause Rickets, osteoporosis, muscle cramps, nervousness, heart palpitations, brittle nails, eczema, hypertension, aching joints, arthritis, tooth decay, insomnia, numbness in the arms and legs, kidney stones, panic attacks, bone spurs, Bell's Palsy, PMS. Causes of depletion: Aspirin, chocolate, stress, lack of exercise, lack of magnesium, lack of hydrochloric acid, high animal protein diet, table salt, excessive phosphorous, oxalic acid, tetracycline, phytic acid.

CATNIP-Has antispasmodic properties, as well as tranquilizing and calming effects. Has some antibiotic properties. Can help ease menstrual cramps. Can help soothe the nerves aiding in a more restful sleep. Can help reduce fever.

CAYENNE-Is a catalysts for all herbs. Helps improve circulation. Aids in digestion. Helps arthritis and rheumatism. Helps stop bleeding ulcers. Good for the kidneys, lungs, pancreas, spleen, heart and stomach.

CHLORINE-Aids in digestion. Helps keep you limber. Regulates the body's electrolyte balance and acid-base balance. Deficiency may cause a loss of hair and teeth.

CHOLINE-Water soluble, a member of the B-complex family and a lipotropic (fat emulsifier). Helps control cholesterol buildup. Aids in the sending of nerve impulses, specifically those in the brain used in the formation of memory. Assists in conquering the problems of memory loss in later years. Aids in the treatment of Alzheimer's disease. Helps eliminate poisons and drugs from your system by aiding the liver. Deficiency may cause cirrhosis and fatty degeneration of liver, hardening of the arteries, and possibly Alzheimer's disease.

CHROMIUM-Aids in growth. Promotes glucose metabolism for energy. Works as a deterrent for diabetes. Helps to prevent and lower high blood pressure. Helps prevent heart attacks. Useful in treating hypoglycemia. Deficiency is a suspected factor in arteriosclerosis and diabetes. Causes of depletion: Refined starches and carbohydrates, sugar.

CHICKWEED-Helps with circulatory problems. May lower blood lipids. Also used for colds, coughs, bronchitis, asthma, skin diseases, and warts.

COBALT-Increases the assimilation of iron. Promotes normal red-blood cell formation. Aids in the assimilation and synthesis of vitamin B12. Stimulates many enzymes for the body. Deficiency may cause anemia. Causes of depletion: Alcohol, sunlight, sleeping pills, estrogen.

COPPER-Required to convert the body's iron into hemoglobin. Keeps you energy up by aiding in effective iron absorption. Converts the amino acid tyrosine that gives color to skin and hair. Involved in the formation of myelin. Promotes normal red-blood cell formation. Promotes connective tissue formation and central nervous system function. Deficiency may cause anemia, edema, skeletal defects and possibly rheumatoid arthritis. Causes of depletion: Excessive zinc and molybdenum.

CRAMP BARK-uterine sedative. Alleviates menstrual cramps.

CYSTEINE-Cysteine helps to detoxify harmful toxins and protects the body from radiation damage. It is one of the best free radical destroyers, and works best when taken with selenium and vitamin E. It helps to protect the liver and brain from damage due to alcohol, drugs, and toxic compounds found in cigarette smoke. Vitamin B6 is necessary for cysteine synthesis. Recommended in the treatment of rheumatoid arthritis, hardening of the arteries, and mutogenic disorders such as cancer. It promotes healing after surgery and severe burns, chelates heavy metals, and binds with soluble iron, aiding in iron absorption. Promotes the burning of fat and the building of muscle. Because of it's ability to break down mucous in the respiratory tract, L-cysteine is often beneficial in the treatment of bronchitis, emphysema, and tuberculosis. It promotes healing from respiratory disorders and plays an important role in the activities of white blood cells, which fight disease. Cysteine aids in preventing side effects from chemotherapy and radiation therapy. It also has an anti-aging effect on the body-reducing the accumulation of age spots, for example. People who have diabetes should be cautious about taking supplemental cysteine because it is capable of inactivating insulin.

DAMIANA-Good for the reproductive organs, nerves, and kidney. Strengthens the male sexual system.

DHEA (Dehydro-Epiandrosterone)-DHEA or Dehydro-Epiandrosterone is a steroid hormone produced in high amounts by the adrenal gland. It is considered the mother of hormones by researchers because it is the precursor of the manufacturing of many other hormones. It is the most abundant steroid in the blood stream. The body produces less DHEA as we age and needs to be supplemented. Can help retard and possibly reverse some of the effects of aging. Helps enhance the immune system. Helps reduce the risk of heart disease. May help stop the effects of carcinogens and reduce the risks of cancer. Aids to promote lean muscle tissue. May increase bone density, reversing the effects of osteoporosis. May help normalize blood sugar levels. Helpful for stress and depression. Also helps with multiple sclerosis and rheumatoid arthritis.

DONG QUAI ROOT-High in vitamin E and iron. Used to dissolve blood clots. Can help to alleviate menopausal hot flashes and depression. Helps alleviate vaginal dryness. Used for all female problems. Increases the effect of ovarian/testicular hormones. During menopause assists in the transition of estrogen production from the ovaries to the adrenal glands.

ECHINACEA-Stimulates the activity of the immune system in general. Protects healthy cells from viral and bacterial attack. Can help lubricate the joints aiding people with arthritis symptoms. Helps fight viruses like colds and influenza. Is a blood cleanser. May help prevent infections by increasing the immune system. Can help preserve white blood counts for patients undergoing radiation treatments (consult with your physician). May help with yeast infections.

ENZYME CO-Q10-Is an enzyme with vitamin-like antioxidant properties that may be more powerful than vitamin E. Levels of coenzyme Q10 decreases with age and should be supplemented. It plays a crucial role in the effectiveness of the immune system and the aging process. All cells have it but it is concentrated in the heart muscle. Studies have shown that a drop in CO-Q10 has caused diseases to flourish. It is essential in the production of energy in every cell in the body. Increases tissue oxygenation. Has been used as treatment for heart disease and high blood pressure. Has benefits to help with the following problems: allergies, asthma, respiratory disease, aging, diabetes, multiple sclerosis, obesity, peridontal disease and candidiasis. May help with mental functions like Alzheimer's disease and schizophrenia. Research is being done to see what benefits it may have for AIDS and cancer. Can possibly reduce side effects of cancer chemotherapy.

FENNEL-Has antispasmodic properties. Can aid with digestive problems. Promotes the functioning of the liver and spleen, and also clears the lungs. Relieves cramping. Can help to promote menstruation. May help to relieve the discomforts of menopause. May help with milk production for nursing mothers. Blood purifier.

FEVER FEW-Has antispasmodic properties. Helps relieve headache pain, including migraines. Helps with dizziness and tinnitus (ringing in the ears). May help reduce blood pressure. Can help with menstrual discomforts. Can help as a digestive aid.

FLOURINE-Reduces tooth decay. Strengthens bones. May prevent and treat osteoporosis. May protect against degenerative disease of the cardiovascular system. Deficiency may cause tooth decay. Causes of depletion: Cooking heat, sugar, aluminum, refined cereals impair the absorption of flourine.

FOLIC ACID-(Folacin, Folate)-Water-soluble. Another member of the B-complex family. Also referred to as Bc or vitamin M. important for the production of nucleic acids DNA and RNA. Essential for the division of body cells. Needed for the utilization of sugar and amino acids. Protects against intestinal parasites and food poisoning. Acts as an analgesic for pain. Helps prevent birth defects. Helps ward off anemia. Improves lactation. Deficiency may cause impaired cell division, anemia, diarrhea, bleeding gums, weight loss, gastrointestinal upsets, irritability.

GARLIC-GARLIC is a natural antibiotic. Protects from infection and detoxifies the body. Garlic is good for all diseases, infections, fungus, and bacteria. To Russians, garlic is known as the "Russian Penicillin" and is considered by some as "The Wonder Drug". Strengthens blood vessels, lowers blood pressure, aids in the treatment of atherosclerosis, asthma, arthritis, cancer, circulatory problems, colds, flu, digestive problems, heart disorders, insomnia, liver disease, sinusitis, ulcers and yeast infections.

GERMANIUM-Helps to fight pain. Keeps the immune system functioning properly. Helps rid the body of toxins and poisons. Increases tissue oxygenation.

GINGER-Has antispasmodic and anti-nausea properties. Can help kill the influenza virus and increases the immune system's ability to fight infection. Has anti-inflammatory properties. Good for morning sickness and motion sickness. Can help with menstrual cramps and hot flashes. Can help fight off colds and flu. Helps with arthritis symptoms. May help prevent heart problems. Can help lower blood pressure and may prevent internal blood clots.

GINKGO BILOBA-Has been called the elixir of long life. Ginkgo products in Europe have sales of over $500 million a year. It has been found to hinder the action of a substance the body produces called platelet aggravation factor (PAF). PAF has been linked to asthma attacks, organ graft rejection, blood clots that cause heart attacks and some strokes. Research is being done for the help with prevention of transplant rejection, and it's effectiveness with allergies, Alzheimer's, and high blood pressure. Can increase blood flow to the brain which can reduce chance of stroke and may help speed recovery from a stroke. Also can improve blood flow to the heart reducing the chance of a heart attack. May help relieve impotence which is caused by lack of blood flow. Improved blood flow to the brain can improve memory. May help with mascular degeneration (an eye disease that causes blindness). Also can help with dizziness (vertigo), hearing damage and tinnitus (ringing in the ears). Can help prevent bronchial constriction, which is helpful for people who have asthma. May also improve blood flow to the legs reducing pain associated with intermittent claudication (narrowing of the arteries). Caution: People with blood clotting problems should use caution when taking Gingko biloba.

GINSENG-There are several forms of ginseng: American, Siberian, Chinese, Korean and Brazilian. There is a slight variation of some of the active chemicals in these different types, overall they have similar effects. Ginseng can have an effect of increased energy. Can stimulate the immune system increasing the ability to fight off viral and bacterial infections. Can help reduce cholesterol and increase good cholesterol

(HDLs), this in turn may reduce the risk of heart attacks. Can help counteract fatigue and increase physical stamina. Can help counteract damage caused by physical and emotional stress. Can also enhance memory. Can reduce blood sugar levels, which can help to manage diabetes. Can help improve liver function and protects the liver from the effects of harmful alcohol or drugs. Can help minimize damage to cancer patients undergoing radiation treatments. Can help as an appetite stimulant and may increase the ability of the intestines to absorb nutrients. Possibly may be a mild sexual stimulant.

GOTU KOLA-Accelerates wound healing, improves circulation in the legs, helps eliminate excess fluids (acts as a diuretic) in the body. Shrinks tissues, stimulates the central nervous system. Increases sex drive. Decreases fatigue and depression. Helps with cardiovascular and circulatory disorders, connective tissue disorders, kidney stones, poor appetite, and sleep disorders.

HOPS-Has properties of being a sedative. May be good for nervousness, pain, stress, insomnia, muscle cramps, toothaches, earaches, and shock. Caution: Pregnant women should not use Hops. Those who have estrogen-dependent breast cancer should use caution when taking this supplement.

IODINE-Promotes proper growth. Is a good antiseptic. Gives you more energy. Promotes healthy hair, nails, skin, and teeth. Protects against toxic effects from radioactive materials. Deficiency may cause goiter and hypothyroidism. Causes of depletion: Heat, food processing.

INOSITOL-Water-soluble, a member of the B-complex family. Aids in redistribution of body fat. Promotes healthy hair-aids in preventing hair fallout. Helps in preventing eczema. Produces a calming effect. Helps in lowering cholesterol levels. Deficiency may cause eczema.

IRON-Aids in growth. Promotes resistance to disease. Prevents fatigue. Can bring back good skin tone. Helps cure and prevent iron-deficiency anemia. Calcium and copper are needed for effective iron absorption. Deficiency may cause iron-deficiency anemia. Causes of depletion: Food additives, preservatives, tea, coffee.

L-ARGININE-Can help with the retardation of tumors and cancer, aids in liver detoxification. Helps release growth hormones and boosts the immune system. Aids in kidney disorders and trauma. Increases sperm count in males. Aids in protein synthesis. Increases muscle mass and reduces body fat. Good for liver disorders. Helps the production of collagen.

L-CARNITINE-Helps transport long-chain fatty acids. Vegetarians are more likely to be deficient in Carnitine due to a diet low in lysine. By helping prevent fatty build-up it aids in weight loss and decreases the risk of heart disease. Can improve athletic ability. Enhances the effectiveness of antioxidants vitamins E & C.

LECITHIN-Lecithin is a type of lipid that is needed by every living cell in the human body. Cell membranes, which regulate the passage of nutrients into and out of the cells, are largely composed of lecithin. The protective sheaths surrounding the brain are composed of lecithin, and the muscles and nerve cells also contain this essential fatty substance. Helps to prevent arteriosclerosis, protects against cardiovascular disease, improves brain function, and aids in the absorption of thiamin by the liver and vitamin A by the intestine. It is also known to promote energy and is needed to help repair damage to the liver caused by alcoholism. Lecithin enables fats, such as cholesterol and other lipids, to be dispersed in water and removed from the body. The vital organs and arteries are thus protected from fatty build-up. Lecithin would be a wise addition to anyone's diet. It is especially valuable for elderly people.

L-GLYCINE-Retards muscle degeneration. Essential for central nervous system function and healthy prostate. Is needed by the immune system to produce the nonessential amino acids. Has inhibitory actions that help prevent epilepsy. Has been used to treat bipolar depression. Proper balance of this amino acid produces more energy. Too much can displace glucose and cause fatigue.

L-HISTIDINE-Essential for the growth and repair of tissues. Histamine is formed from histidine and is usually released by the cells as a immune response. Needed for the treatment of allergies, rheumatoid arthritis, and anemia. Aids in the production of red and white blood cells. Aids in digestive problems: ulcers, hyperacidity, gastric juices and general digestion.

LICORICE ROOT-Has anti-inflammatory and arthritic properties. It stimulates cell production of interferon, (the body's antiviral compound). Has properties to fight disease-causing bacteria and the fungus responsible for vaginal yeast infections (Candida albicans). Can help as a stimulant for intestinal secretion to help as a treatment for ulcers. Has been used to treat liver problems and help control hepatitis. May be beneficial for hypoglycemia, bronchitis, stress, colds, nausea, colitis, and inflammation. May decrease muscle or skeletal spasms. Caution: People with high blood pressure, diabetes, glaucoma, or a history of heart disease should use caution when taking licorice root. Pregnant women should not use it.

L-ISOLEUCINE-Needed for the formation of hemoglobin. It is metabolized in muscle tissues. Should be taken with the correct balance of leucine and valine. Helps regulate blood sugar and energy levels. Deficiency can lead to symptoms similar to those of hypoglycemia (low blood sugar).

L-LEUCINE-Should be taken in balance with isoleucine and valine. Should be taken in moderation, or hypoglycemia may result. Lowers elevated blood sugar levels. Promotes the healing of bone, skin, and muscle tissue. Is recommended for those recovering from surgery.

L-LYSINE-Lysine is an essential amino acid that is a necessary building block for all protein. Aids in the production of antibodies, hormones and enzymes. Aids in the production of collagen and the repair of tissues. Needed for proper growth and bone development in children. Aids in the absorption of calcium and helps to maintain the nitrogen balance in adults. Aids in fighting viruses like cold sores and Herpes. Important for those recovering from surgery and sports injuries. Lowers high serum triglycerides. Deficiencies result in loss of energy, inability to concentrate, irritability, anemia, retarded growth and reproduction disorders, hair loss and blood shot eyes.

MAGNESIUM-Essential for effective nerve and muscle functioning. Important for converting blood sugar into energy. Aids in fighting depression. Needed for healthy bones. Helps to keep your cardiovascular system healthier and helps to prevent heart attacks. May reduce blood pressure. Helps prevent calcium deposits, kidney stones and gallstones. Magnesium is a brain and nerve food element stored in combination with Lecithin. Required for the formation of red-blood cells. Deficiency may cause muscle weakness, twitching, cramps, cardiac disturbances, menstrual migraines, depression, asthma, anorexia, vertigo. Causes of depletion: Alcohol, diuretics, coffee, tobacco, refined sugar, digitalis medications.

MARSHMALLOW ROOT-Soothes and heals skin, mucous membranes, and other tissues, externally and internally. Acts as a diuretic and expectorant. May help relieve upset stomach. May help with the respiratory rawness associated with sore throat, cough, colds, flu, and bronchitis. May help boost the immune system to help fight infections.

MANGANESE-Needed for normal bone structure. Needed for the formation of thyroxin, a hormone of the thyroid gland. Aids in the digestion of utilization of food. Helps in reproduction functioning and normal nervous system function. Reduces nervous irritability. Essential for the proper functioning of the pituitary gland. Deficiency may cause muscular and mental fatigue. Causes of depletion: Large phosphorous and calcium intake, also a high iron intake.

MELATONIN-Is a naturally occurring hormone whose primary function is to promote sleep. Middle age adults (45) secrete only half as much as children and at age 80 production slows to a trickle. It helps correct the disordered circadian rhythms of jet lag and shift work. Helps with mood swings. Melatonin also has very good antioxidant properties.

MOLYBDENUM-Essential for enzyme actions. Believed to help prevent esophageal cancer and dental carries. Frees iron stored in the liver carrying oxygen to body cells and tissues. Helps eliminate toxic nitrogen waste. Deficiency may cause anemia. Causes of depletion: Copper and refined foods.

PASSION FLOWER-Contains substances that have the properties of being a tranquilizer or mild sedative. Has antispasmodic properties. Used as a tranquilizer or mild sedative. May help as a digestive aid. May help with menstrual cramps. May help kill bacteria, mold, and fungi; aiding as a wound treatment. May help relieve pain.

PEPPERMINT-Peppermint is an antispasmodic and stimulant. Increases stomach acidity. Has anti-inflammatory and antiarthritic properties. Fights disease-causing bacteria and the fungus that causes vaginal yeast infections. Used for heart trouble, rheumatism, convulsions, spasms, headaches, chills, colic, fever, nausea and diarrhea. Helps control hepatitis and improves liver functions.

PHENYLALANINE-Promotes alertness, elevates mood, decreases pain, aids in memory and learning, and increases appetite. Can be used to treat arthritis, depression, menstrual cramps, migraines, obesity, Parkinson's disease, and schizophrenia. Caution: Supplemental phenylalanine should not be taken by PREGNANT WOMEN or by people who suffer from anxiety attacks, flu, high blood pressure, phenylketonuria (PKU), or pre-existing melanoma.

PHOSPHOROUS-Present in every cell in the body. Involved in virtually all physiological chemical reactions. Important for heart regularity. Essential for normal kidney functioning. Needed for the transference of nerve impulses. Provides energy and vigor by helping in the metabolism of fats and starches. Lessens the pain of arthritis. Necessary for healthy bones. Essential for cell division and replication. Stimulates blood circulation. Deficiency may cause Rickets, pyorrhea. Causes of depletion: Sugar, tobacco, mineral oil, excess intake of aluminum, magnesium and iron, salts from cookware.

POTASSIUM-Aids in clear thinking by sending oxygen to the brain. Aids in regulating the body's water balance. Main healing mineral. Protective against stroke. Assists in reducing blood pressure. Improves anti-cancer cells. Aids in nerve and muscle functions. Deficiency may cause edema, hypoglycemia, cardiac disturbances such as irregular heartbeat, irritability, muscle weakness. Causes of depletion: Cooking and processing, alcohol, coffee, diuretics, laxatives, cortisone, excess salt.

PRIMROSE OIL-Contains highest amount of GLA (gamma-linolenic acid) an essential fatty acid. GLA is needed to produce hormone like compounds called prostaglandins (PGs) which are vital for good health. A deficiency of GLA can result in impaired production of PGs and adversely effect your physical well-being. Can help to lower cholesterol levels and high blood pressure. Aids in weight loss, menstrual disorders, relieves hot flashes, helps with skin disorders, multiple sclerosis, and arthritic pain. Caution: Those suffering from estrogen related breast cancer should limit their intake of primrose oil.

PROANTHOCYANIDINS (pycnogenol: grape seed extract, pine bark extract)-Proanthocyanidin is a naturally occurring bioflavonoid in a wide variety of plants, however, the main two sources are from pine bark extract and grape seed extract. Proanthocyanidin is a unique flavonol and an extremely powerful antioxidant, that is 50 times more potent than vitamin E and 20 times more potent than vitamin C. It helps protect and boost the effectiveness of other nutrients so they work better. Reduces the risk of heart disease, cancer, accelerated aging, oxidative stress, arthritis, and more than 70 other radical-related diseases. Strengthens blood vessels and reduces capillary fragility, reduces bruising, reduces the severity of sports injuries, reduces varicose veins, reduces edema and the swelling of the legs, treats chronic venous insufficiency, and reduces the risk of phlebitis. Improves red-blood-cell membrane flexibility. Improves skin elasticity and smoothness. Protects against sun damage. Effective against psoriasis. Very effective against hay fever. Helps reduce inflammation.

Improves joint flexibility. Reduces the pain due to swollen joints. Reduces diabetic retinopathy. Enhances immune response. Reduces the frequency and severity of colds. Reduces retinopathies. Helps prevent capillary bleeding, floaters. Helps with Alzheimer's. reduces the risk of Parkinson's. Acts against stomach ulcers and inflammation. Many diseases are related to free radical damage. Proanthocyanidin crosses the blood-brain barrier and promotes healing within the brain. This is the only product available without a prescription that is able to do this. This is why it is so effecting in treating disorders of the brain such as Alzheimer's disease and Attention Deficit Disorder.

RED CLOVER-A sweet herb that is a blood purifier, an antibiotic used for tuberculosis and to fight other bacteria. A relaxant and an appetite suppressant. May help relieve menopausal symptoms. There are claims that it may help with non-estrogen cancer tumors. Good for inflamed lungs, whooping cough, and other inflammatory conditions related to gout and arthritis. Can help with skin disorders. Caution: Those who have cancers aggravated by estrogen should use caution when using red clover.

ROSEHIPS-Good source of vitamin C. Helps for colds and flu. Good for infections and bladder problems. Helps combat stress.

ROSEMARY-Because of the very powerful antioxidant properties, it has very strong preservative powers, compares with commercial food preservatives, BHA and BHT. Good as a digestive aid. Helps relieve nasal and chest congestion from colds and allergies. Has antispasmodic properties.

SAGE—Because of the very powerful antioxidant properties, it has very strong preservative powers, compares with commercial food preservatives, BHA and BHT. Good as a digestive aid. May help to promote menstrual cycle. May help with wound healing by preventing infections. May help with sore throat. Has antispasmodic properties.

SASPARILLA-Helps regulate hormones. Is a good blood purifier. Acts as a diuretic. Increases energy. May be good for stomach and kidney problems. Has been used as treatment for impotence, liver problems, rheumatism, and gout. May reduce fever and clear up skin disorders.

SAW PALMETTEO-Acts as a diuretic and urinary antiseptic. May enhance sexual functioning and desire. Stimulates appetite. Helps inhibit production of the hormone that causes enlargement of the prostate.

SCULLCAP-Excellent for almost any nervous system malfunction. Aids in weaning individuals from barbiturate addiction and excessive use of valium. Helps as a sedative, nerve tonic, and antispasmodic. Improves circulation and strengthens heart muscle. Helps to strengthen and support the nervous system. Helps for a wide range of nervous disorders, insomnia, anxiety, and digestive problems. Relieves pain, stress, muscle cramps, and spasms.

SELENIUM-Synergistic with vitamin E-also an antioxidant. Aids in keeping youthful elasticity in tissues. Alleviates hot flashes and menopausal distress. Helps in the treatment and prevention of dandruff. Possibly can neutralize certain carcinogens and provides protection from certain cancers, especially breast cancer. Helps to prevent chromosome breakage causing birth defects. Deficiency may cause HIV, Cardiomyopathy, anemia, age spots, fatigue, myalgia, Scoliosis, Cystic Fibrosis, infertility, SIDS, Alzheimer's disease, irregular heart beat. Causes of depletion: High fat intake, stress.

SILICON (Silica)-Necessary for bone and connective tissue (collagen) formation for healthy hair, skin, and nails. Aids in calcium absorption and bone formation. Counteracts the effects of aluminum aiding in the prevention of Alzheimer's disease and osteoporosis. Is needed to maintain flexible arteries and helps prevent cardiovascular disease. Increases the alkalinity of the body. Essential for healthy blood cells and proper blood circulation. Deficiency may cause mental fatigue, baldness, nervousness, exhaustion. Causes of depletion: Fats, starches, and sugar.

SLIPPERY ELM BARK-Contains B-complex vitamins and is high in protein. Has beneficial effects on the entire body. Helps heal and soothe inflamed or irritated areas. Helps with cough, sore throat, diarrhea, ulcers, colitis, vaginal irritations, and hemorrhoids. Neutralizes stomach acidity and absorbs noxious gases.

SODIUM-Aids in preventing heat prostration or sunstroke. Helps your nerves and muscles function properly. Plays a crucial role in maintaining blood pressure. Prevents arthritis. Helps regulate the water balance in the body. Regulates the body's acid-base balance. Deficiency may cause impaired carbohydrate digestion, possibly neuralgia, and in severe cases a decrease in the level of cognitive functioning. Causes of depletion: Diarrhea, exercise, hot climate, sweating, vomiting.

SPIRULINA-Recognized as the most promising of all microalgae. Is being considered as an immediate food source. It produces 20 times the amount of protein as that of soybeans on an equal land area.

Contains high amounts of vitamin B12, has a 60-70 percent protein content, high iron content, essential amino acids, RNA and DNA nucleic acids, chlorophyll, and blue pigment (phycocyanin) found only in green-blue algae, which may help with fighting cancer. Aids in protecting the immune system, lowering cholesterol, and in mineral absorption. Helps to cleanse and heal. May help reduce appetite. Good for hypoglycemia because it's high protein content helps to stabilize blood sugar levels.

SULFUR-Essential for healthy hair, skin, and nails. Helps fight bacterial infections. Helps maintain oxygen balance necessary for proper brain functioning. Known as a beauty mineral. Essential for protein absorption. Works with B-complex vitamins. Causes of depletion: Cooking.

THREONINE-Threonine is an important amino acid that helps to maintain the proper protein balance in the body. It is important for the formation of collagen and elastin. Threonine is present in the heart, central nervous system and skeletal muscle, and helps to prevent fatty buildup in the liver. It enhances the immune system by aiding in the production of antibodies.

VALERIAN ROOT-Valerian root is nourishing and soothing to the nervous system. Helps as a sedative for nervousness, anxiety, stress, and hysteria. Improves circulation. May also help with colds, coughs, migraines, muscle pains, cramps, insomnia, high blood pressure, headaches, and chest congestion.

VALINE-Valine is an essential amino acid and has a stimulant effect. It is needed for muscle metabolism, tissue repair, and the maintenance of a proper nitrogen balance in the body. Valine is found in high concentrations in muscle tissue. It is one of the branch-chained amino acids, which means that it can be used as an energy source by muscle tissue. It is good for correcting the severe type of amino acid deficiencies that can be caused by drug addiction. An excessively high level of valine may lead to such symptoms as a crawling sensation in the skin and even hallucinations.

VANADIUM-Inhibits the formation of cholesterol in blood vessels. Aids in preventing heart attacks. Essential for proper circulation. Essential in iron-metabolism. Plays a role in the metabolism of bones and teeth. Plays a role in energy production. Deficiency may cause sugar cravings. Causes of depletion: food processing.

WHITE OAK BARK-Contains the nutrients calcium, manganese, iodine, iron, magnesium, selenium, potassium, silicon, and zinc. Is good for skin, teeth, kidneys, varicose veins, Herpes, thrush, and yeast infections. Contains properties for clotting, shrinking, and disinfecting.

WHITE WILLOW BARK-Contains the chemical that aspirin is derived from. Good as a pain reliever for headaches, arthritis, menstrual cramps, and other pains and inflammations.

WOOD BETONY-Contains the nutrients magnesium, manganese, phosphorous, and tannins. Stimulates the heart and relaxes the muscles. Acts as a mild sedative to the central nervous system. Good for the immune system, nerves, liver and spleen.

ZINC-Essential for protein synthesis. Helps in the formation of insulin. Important for blood stability and in maintaining the body's acid-alkaline balance. Essential for the growth of children's bones and teeth. Maintains normal taste and smell. Maintains normal levels of vitamin A in the blood. Accelerates healing time for internal and external wounds. Kills Rhinovirus, when absorbed orally, on contact. Rhinovirus is one of the more than 200 different cold viruses that give us the common cold. Aids in the treatment of infertility. Helps avoid prostate problems. Promotes growth and mental alertness. Helps decrease cholesterol deposits. Aids in the treatment of mental disorders. Deficiency may cause a loss of taste or smell, Down's syndrome, cleft lip, spina bifida, infertility, failure of wounds to heal, poor growth, hair loss, anorexia, or bulimia. Causes of depletion: Excessive calcium, antacids, alcohol, oral contraceptives.

Compiled and researched by;
Velvet Fitzsimmons
Former registed nurse